The Cancer Prevention Handbook:

Practical Strategies for Lowering Your Risk

By

Ismael A. Fisher

Table of Contents

Specific Types of Physical Activity for Cancer Prevention.
Strategies for Maintaining Regular Physical Activity.
Physical Activity and Cancer Survivorship.

Environmental Factors and Cancer Prevention
Chemicals and Cancer Risk.
Air Pollution and Cancer Risk.
Radiation and Cancer Risk.
Practical Strategies for Reducing Environmental Exposures and Lowering Cancer Risk.

Lifestyle Factors and Cancer Prevention
Diet and Cancer Risk.
Physical Activity and Cancer Risk.
Tobacco and Alcohol Use and Cancer Risk

<u>Chapter 8:</u>

Cancer Screening and Early Detection

Introduction

Cancer. The very word strikes fear into the hearts of many. It's a disease that has touched the lives of almost everyone in some way, whether through personal experience or the experience of a loved one. But did you know that there are simple steps you can take to lower your risk of developing cancer?

In this book, we'll explore the latest scientific research and evidence-based strategies for cancer prevention. From lifestyle changes to dietary habits, we'll cover it all. You'll learn about the foods that can help lower your cancer risk, as well as the foods that you should avoid. We'll discuss the role of exercise in cancer prevention, and how to make it a part of your daily routine.

But cancer prevention is about more than just diet and exercise. We'll also delve into the importance of stress reduction, sleep hygiene, and avoiding environmental toxins. We'll examine the latest research on supplements and alternative therapies, and what you can do to make informed choices about your health.

The goal of this book is simple: to empower you with the knowledge and tools you need to take control of your health and reduce your risk of developing cancer. Whether you're looking to make small changes to your daily routine or are ready for a complete lifestyle overhaul, this book is for you. So let's get started on the path to a healthier, cancer-free life.

Throughout this book, we'll draw on the expertise of leading cancer researchers, oncologists, and nutritionists to bring you the most up-to-date and accurate information available. But we'll also make it accessible and easy to understand, so you don't need a medical degree to benefit from this knowledge.

It's important to remember that while cancer can be a daunting and frightening topic, there is hope. Research shows that up to 50% of all cancers are preventable through lifestyle changes alone. This means that by making simple changes to our diet, exercise habits, and daily routines, we can dramatically reduce our risk of developing cancer.

But it's not just about preventing cancer. By adopting a healthier lifestyle, we can also improve our overall health and wellbeing. We'll explore how small changes in our daily routine can have a big impact on our health, from reducing inflammation to boosting our immune system.

Whether you're looking to prevent cancer, improve your health, or simply learn more about this complex disease, "The Cancer

Prevention Handbook: Practical Strategies for Lowering Your Risk" is the ultimate guide to achieving your goals. So let's begin the journey towards a healthier, happier life.

Chapter 1:

Understanding Cancer Risk Factors

Cancer is a complex disease that arises from the uncontrolled growth and spread of abnormal cells in the body. There are many different types of cancer, each with their unique characteristics, risk factors, and treatment options. In this explanation, we will focus on some of the most common types of cancer, including breast, lung, prostate, and colon cancer, and provide an overview of how cancer forms and spreads, the definition of risk factors, and how they contribute to cancer development.

Breast Cancer:

Breast cancer is a type of cancer that forms in the breast tissue. It is the most common cancer in women worldwide and can also affect men. Breast cancer typically forms in the milk ducts or lobules of the breast and can spread to nearby lymph nodes and other parts of the body. Risk factors for breast cancer include age, family history, certain gene mutations, exposure to radiation, obesity, and alcohol consumption.

Lung Cancer:

Lung cancer is a type of cancer that forms in the lungs, typically in the cells that line the airways. It is the leading cause of cancer-related deaths worldwide and is often caused by smoking or exposure to second-hand smoke. Other risk factors for lung cancer include exposure to radon, asbestos, and other chemicals and pollutants.

Prostate Cancer:

Prostate cancer is a type of cancer that forms in the prostate gland, which is located below the bladder in men. It is one of the most common types of cancer in men and usually develops slowly over many years. Risk factors for prostate cancer include age, family history, and certain gene mutations.

Colon Cancer:

Colon cancer is a type of cancer that forms in the colon or rectum. It typically starts as a small growth called a polyp that can become cancerous over time. Risk factors for colon cancer include age, family history, a history of polyps or inflammatory bowel disease, and a diet high in red and processed meats.

Other Types of Cancer:

There are many other types of cancer, including skin cancer, ovarian cancer, pancreatic cancer, and leukemia, among others. Each type of cancer has its unique risk factors, symptoms, and treatment options.

Cancer Formation and Spread:

Cancer forms when the DNA in a cell is damaged, causing it to divide and grow uncontrollably. Over time, these abnormal cells can form a mass or tumor, which can invade nearby tissues and spread to other parts of the body through the bloodstream or lymphatic system. The spread of cancer is called metastasis and can make treatment more difficult.

Risk Factors and Cancer Development:

Risk factors are things that increase a person's chances of developing cancer. Some risk factors, such as age and family history, cannot be changed, while others, such as smoking and diet, can be modified to reduce cancer risk. Other risk factors for cancer include exposure to radiation, certain chemicals and pollutants, and viruses and bacteria.

Cancer is a complex disease that can arise from a combination of various risk factors. These risk factors can be divided into four main categories: age, genetics, environmental factors, and lifestyle factors. In this explanation, we will provide an overview of these common cancer risk factors and how they contribute to cancer development.

Age:

Age is one of the most significant risk factors for cancer. As people age, the risk of developing cancer increases. This is because the accumulation of genetic mutations and environmental exposures over time can lead to the development of cancer.

Genetics:

Some people may be genetically predisposed to developing cancer. Inherited genetic mutations can increase the risk of developing certain types of cancer, such as breast, ovarian, and colon cancer. Genetic testing can help identify individuals who may be at higher risk for cancer due to inherited mutations.

Environmental Factors:

Environmental factors, such as exposure to radiation, chemicals, and pollutants, can increase the risk of cancer. Exposure to certain chemicals, such as asbestos and benzene, is known to increase the risk of developing lung cancer and leukemia, respectively. Exposure to ultraviolet radiation from the sun can increase the risk of skin cancer.

Lifestyle Factors:

Lifestyle factors, such as tobacco use, poor diet, lack of physical activity, and alcohol consumption, can also increase the risk of cancer. Smoking is the leading cause of lung cancer and is responsible for a significant proportion of other cancer types as well. A diet high in red and processed meats can increase the risk of colon cancer. Lack of physical activity and obesity are also known to increase the risk of various types of cancer.

Multiple Risk Factors:

It is important to note that cancer risk is not solely determined by one risk factor but rather by a combination of factors. For example, an individual who smokes and is exposed to asbestos has a higher risk of developing lung cancer than someone who only smokes or is only exposed to asbestos. Multiple risk factors can interact and increase the likelihood of cancer development.

In conclusion, understanding the common cancer risk factors, including age, genetics, environmental factors, and lifestyle factors, is critical in reducing cancer risk and improving outcomes. By identifying and modifying these risk factors, individuals can reduce their chances of developing cancer and increase their chances of successful treatment if cancer does develop.

Genetics and Family History of Cancer

Inherited genetic mutations can increase the risk of developing cancer. These mutations are changes in the DNA sequence that are passed down from parents to their offspring. Inherited mutations can alter the function of specific genes that regulate cell growth and division, leading to an increased risk of developing cancer.

Common Genetic Mutations:

There are several genetic mutations that have been linked to an increased risk of developing cancer. Two of the most well-known mutations are BRCA1 and BRCA2. These genes normally produce proteins that help suppress the growth of tumors. However, when mutations occur in these genes, the proteins produced are not able to perform their tumor-suppressing functions effectively, increasing the risk of developing breast and ovarian cancer in women, and prostate cancer in men. Other genetic mutations associated with increased cancer risk include APC, TP53, and Lynch syndrome.

Family History:

Family history is another important factor in assessing an individual's risk of developing cancer. If multiple family members have been diagnosed with cancer, especially at a young age, it may indicate the presence of an inherited genetic mutation. Individuals with a family history of cancer should consider genetic counseling and testing to determine if they carry a genetic mutation that increases their cancer risk.

Genetic Counseling:

Genetic counseling is a process in which a trained professional helps individuals understand their risk of developing cancer based on their family history and personal medical history. Genetic counseling involves assessing an individual's risk of developing cancer, discussing the benefits and limitations of genetic testing, and developing a personalized prevention and screening plan based on the results of genetic testing.

Genetic counseling can help individuals make informed decisions about their healthcare and take proactive steps to reduce their risk of developing cancer. It can also provide peace of mind to individuals who have concerns about their family history and want to better understand their risk of developing cancer.

In conclusion, inherited genetic mutations can significantly increase an individual's risk of developing cancer. Understanding one's family history and undergoing genetic counseling and testing can help identify genetic mutations and inform personalized prevention and screening strategies. Early detection and prevention are crucial in reducing cancer risk and improving outcomes, and genetic counseling can play an important role in achieving these goals.

Environmental Factors and Cancer Risk

Environmental factors play a significant role in cancer development. Exposure to certain substances and conditions in the environment can increase cancer risk. Some common environmental factors that can increase cancer risk include exposure to tobacco smoke, air pollution, and hazardous chemicals.

Tobacco smoke contains carcinogens, chemicals that can cause cancer. Smoking is the leading cause of lung cancer and is also associated with several other types of cancer, including bladder, kidney, and pancreatic cancer. Exposure to secondhand smoke can also increase cancer risk.

Air pollution is another environmental factor that can increase cancer risk. Exposure to pollutants in the air, such as particulate matter, can cause inflammation in the body and damage DNA, which can lead to cancer. Air pollution has been linked to lung cancer, as well as other types of cancer, such as bladder cancer.

Exposure to hazardous chemicals in the workplace can also increase cancer risk. Workers in certain industries, such as manufacturing, construction, and agriculture, may be exposed to chemicals that are known to cause cancer. For example, exposure to asbestos, a mineral that was commonly used in building materials until the 1970s, is a known cause of lung cancer and mesothelioma, a cancer of the lining of the lungs.

Exposure to radiation is another environmental factor that can increase cancer risk. Radiation can damage DNA, which can lead to the development of cancer. Exposure to high levels of radiation, such as from nuclear accidents or radiation therapy for cancer treatment, can increase cancer risk.

In conclusion, environmental factors play a significant role in cancer development. Exposure to tobacco smoke, air pollution, hazardous chemicals, and radiation can increase cancer risk. It is important to reduce exposure to these factors whenever possible, through measures such as quitting smoking, reducing air pollution, and using protective equipment in the workplace.

Lifestyle Factors and Cancer Risk

Lifestyle factors are also significant contributors to cancer development. Poor diet, lack of exercise, and chronic stress are some of the lifestyle factors that can increase cancer risk.

A poor diet that is high in processed and sugary foods, red meat, and saturated fat, and low in fruits, vegetables, and whole grains, can increase inflammation and oxidative stress in the body, which can contribute to cancer development. In contrast, a healthy diet that is rich in plant-based foods, lean protein, and healthy fats can help reduce inflammation and oxidative stress and lower cancer risk.

Lack of exercise is another lifestyle factor that can increase cancer risk. Regular physical activity can help reduce inflammation and oxidative stress in the body, as well as promote healthy hormone levels, which can help lower cancer risk. In contrast, a sedentary lifestyle can increase inflammation and oxidative stress and contribute to cancer development.

Chronic stress is also a lifestyle factor that can increase cancer risk. Prolonged stress can lead to chronic inflammation and oxidative stress in the body, which can contribute to cancer development. Stress management techniques, such as meditation, yoga, and relaxation exercises, can help reduce stress and lower cancer risk.

In addition to inflammation and oxidative stress, lifestyle factors can also affect hormone levels, which can increase cancer risk in certain types of cancer. For example, in breast cancer and prostate cancer, higher levels of estrogen and testosterone, respectively, can increase cancer risk.

Lifestyle factors that can affect hormone levels, such as obesity, lack of exercise, and alcohol consumption, can increase cancer risk in these types of cancer.

Factors play a significant role in cancer development. Poor diet, lack of exercise, and chronic stress can increase inflammation and oxidative stress, while also affecting hormone levels, which can contribute to cancer development. It is important to adopt healthy lifestyle habits, such as a healthy diet, regular exercise, and stress management techniques, to help reduce cancer risk.

Chapter 2:

Nutrition and Cancer Prevention

The role of diet in cancer prevention is crucial. Certain dietary patterns can increase or decrease cancer risk. A diet that is high in plant-based foods, such as fruits, vegetables, whole grains, legumes, and nuts, and low in processed and sugary foods, red meat, and saturated fat, has been associated with a lower risk of cancer.

One reason for this is that plant-based foods are rich in nutrients that can help protect against cancer development. For example, antioxidants, such as vitamins C and E, beta-carotene, and selenium, can help protect cells from damage that can lead to cancer. Phytochemicals, such as flavonoids and carotenoids, can also help protect against cancer development by reducing inflammation and oxidative stress in the body.

On the other hand, a diet that is high in processed and sugary foods, red meat, and saturated fat, can increase cancer risk. These foods have been linked to inflammation and oxidative stress in the body, which can contribute to cancer development.

In addition to specific nutrients, the overall dietary pattern is also important for cancer prevention. For example, the Mediterranean diet, which is high in plant-based foods, healthy fats, and lean protein, has been associated with a lower risk of cancer. The DASH diet, which is high in fruits, vegetables, whole grains, and lean protein, and low in sodium and saturated fat, has also been associated with a lower risk of cancer.

In summary, the role of diet in cancer prevention is crucial. A diet that is high in plant-based foods, such as fruits, vegetables, whole grains, legumes, and nuts, and low in processed and sugary foods, red meat, and saturated fat, has been associated with a lower risk of cancer. Nutrients such as antioxidants and phytochemicals can help protect against cancer development, while a diet high in processed and sugary foods, red meat, and saturated fat can increase cancer risk. Adopting a healthy dietary pattern, such as the Mediterranean diet or DASH diet, can help reduce cancer risk.

Foods That Can Lower Your Risk of Cancer

Research has shown that certain foods can play a role in cancer prevention. These foods are typically nutrient-dense, high in antioxidants, and have anti-inflammatory properties. Here are some specific foods that have been linked to cancer prevention:

Fruits and vegetables: A diet rich in fruits and vegetables has been linked to a lower risk of many types of cancer. These foods are high in fiber, vitamins, and minerals, as well as phytochemicals that can help protect against cancer development. Some specific types of fruits and vegetables that have been linked to lower cancer risk include cruciferous vegetables (such as broccoli, cauliflower, and Brussels sprouts), berries (such as blueberries and raspberries), and leafy green vegetables (such as spinach and kale).

Whole grains: Whole grains are an important source of fiber and other nutrients that can help protect against cancer. Studies have shown that a diet rich in whole grains can lower the risk of colorectal cancer.

Legumes: Legumes, such as beans, lentils, and chickpeas, are a good source of protein and fiber, as well as other nutrients that can help protect against cancer. Research has linked a higher intake of legumes with a lower risk of colorectal cancer.

Nuts and seeds: Nuts and seeds are high in healthy fats, protein, and fiber, as well as antioxidants that can help protect against cancer. Some specific types of nuts and seeds that have been linked to lower cancer risk include walnuts, almonds, and flaxseeds.

These foods contain a variety of nutrients that can help protect against cancer development, including antioxidants (such as vitamin C and beta-carotene), fiber, and phytochemicals (such as resveratrol and quercetin). Antioxidants can help protect against damage to DNA that can lead to cancer development. Fiber can help lower the risk of colorectal cancer by promoting regular bowel movements and helping to eliminate carcinogens from the body. Phytochemicals have anti-inflammatory properties that can help reduce the risk of cancer.

Overall, a diet rich in fruits, vegetables, whole grains, legumes, nuts, and seeds can help lower cancer risk. It is important to eat a variety of these foods to ensure that you are getting a range of nutrients that can help protect against cancer.

Foods to Avoid or Limit for Cancer Prevention

Certain foods and nutrients have been linked to an increased risk of developing cancer. These foods and nutrients can contribute to cancer development by increasing inflammation and oxidative stress in the body, which can lead to DNA damage and the formation of cancerous cells.

Red and processed meats are one of the most well-known dietary factors that have been linked to increased cancer risk. The consumption of these meats has been shown to increase the risk of colon, stomach, and prostate cancer. The high levels of saturated and trans fats found in these meats are thought to contribute to cancer development by promoting inflammation in the body.

Similarly, diets high in saturated and trans fats, such as those found in fried foods and baked goods, have also been linked to an increased risk of certain types of cancer. These fats can increase oxidative stress and inflammation in the body, leading to the development of cancerous cells.

Excess alcohol consumption has also been linked to an increased risk of cancer, particularly in the liver, breast, and colon. Alcohol can increase oxidative stress in the body and damage DNA, leading to the formation of cancer cells.

It is important to limit or avoid these foods and nutrients to lower the risk of cancer. Instead, focus on a diet rich in fruits, vegetables, whole grains, legumes, nuts, and seeds, which have been shown to have cancer-fighting properties. By making these dietary changes, you can help reduce your risk of developing cancer and promote overall health and wellbeing.

The Importance of Maintaining a Healthy Weight for Cancer Prevention

Excess body weight is a well-established risk factor for various types of cancer, including breast, colon, and prostate cancer. When the body carries excess fat, it produces higher levels of hormones and inflammatory molecules, which can lead to DNA damage and promote cancer development. Additionally, fat tissue can produce insulin resistance and high insulin levels, which can also increase cancer risk.

Maintaining a healthy weight through a healthy diet and regular exercise can help lower cancer risk. A healthy diet should include plenty of fruits, vegetables, whole grains, and lean proteins, while limiting processed and high-fat foods. Portion control is also important to prevent overeating and weight gain. Regular physical activity, such as brisk walking, cycling, or swimming, can help burn calories, strengthen muscles, and improve overall health.

Stress management can also play a role in maintaining a healthy weight and reducing cancer risk. Chronic stress can lead to overeating and weight gain, so finding healthy ways to manage stress, such as yoga, meditation, or counseling, can be beneficial. Additionally, getting adequate sleep and avoiding smoking can also help lower cancer risk.

Specific strategies for achieving and maintaining a healthy weight include setting realistic goals, tracking food intake and exercise, finding support from friends or family, and seeking guidance from a healthcare professional or registered dietitian. By adopting a healthy lifestyle and maintaining a healthy weight, individuals can lower their cancer risk and improve overall health.

Chapter 3:

Physical Activity and Cancer Prevention

Physical activity has been found to be an effective strategy for cancer prevention. There is a link between physical activity and cancer prevention, with numerous studies indicating that physical activity can lower the risk of developing certain types of cancer. The mechanism behind this link is multifactorial, and several mechanisms have been proposed to explain the association between physical activity and cancer prevention.

One way in which physical activity can lower cancer risk is by reducing inflammation and oxidative stress. Chronic inflammation and oxidative stress are known to play a key role in cancer development, and physical activity has been found to reduce both of these factors. When we engage in physical activity, our body produces antioxidants that counteract oxidative stress and reduce inflammation, which can help prevent cancer.

In addition, physical activity can also promote healthy hormone levels. Some hormones, such as estrogen, have been linked to an increased risk of certain types of cancer. Regular physical activity can help regulate hormone levels, which can reduce the risk of developing cancer.

Physical activity can also support a healthy immune system, which is important for cancer prevention. When we exercise, our immune system produces more white blood cells, which can help fight off cancer cells and other diseases.

The types and amounts of physical activity recommended for cancer prevention vary depending on the individual's age, health status, and fitness level. Generally, adults should aim for at least 150 minutes of moderate-intensity aerobic activity per week, or 75 minutes of vigorous-intensity aerobic activity per week. Strength training exercises should also be performed at least twice a week.

Examples of moderate-intensity aerobic activities include brisk walking, cycling, and swimming. Examples of vigorous-intensity aerobic activities include running, cycling at a high intensity, and high-intensity interval training (HIIT). Strength training exercises can include weightlifting, bodyweight exercises, and resistance band exercises.

In summary, physical activity can lower the risk of developing certain types of cancer by reducing inflammation and oxidative stress, promoting healthy hormone levels, and supporting a healthy immune system. The types and amounts of physical activity recommended for cancer prevention vary depending on the individual, but generally, adults should aim for at least 150 minutes of moderate-intensity aerobic activity per week, along with strength training exercises at least twice a week.

Specific Types of Physical Activity for Cancer Prevention

There are several types of physical activity that have been linked to lower cancer risk, including moderate-intensity aerobic activity, strength training, and flexibility exercises. Each type of physical activity can provide different benefits for cancer prevention.

Moderate-intensity aerobic activity, such as brisk walking, cycling, and swimming, has been found to lower the risk of several types of cancer, including breast, colon, and lung cancer. This type of exercise can help reduce inflammation, improve insulin sensitivity, and regulate hormone levels, all of which can contribute to a lower risk of cancer.

Strength training exercises, such as weightlifting, bodyweight exercises, and resistance band exercises, can help improve muscle mass and strength, which can improve overall health and reduce the risk of certain types of cancer, including breast and colon cancer. Strength training exercises can also help regulate hormone levels and reduce inflammation, which can contribute to a lower risk of cancer.

Flexibility exercises, such as yoga and stretching, can help improve range of motion and flexibility, which can reduce the risk of injury during other types of exercise. In addition, flexibility exercises can help reduce stress, which can also contribute to a lower risk of cancer.

To incorporate different types of physical activity into a comprehensive exercise plan for cancer prevention, it is important to consider the individual's preferences, fitness level, and overall health status. It is recommended to engage in at least 150 minutes of moderate-intensity aerobic activity per week, along with strength training exercises at least twice a week and flexibility exercises on a regular basis.

One way to incorporate these different types of physical activity into an exercise plan is to alternate between different types of exercise throughout the week. For example, one day could be dedicated to moderate-intensity aerobic activity, another day could be dedicated to strength training exercises, and a third day could be dedicated to flexibility exercises.

Another way to incorporate different types of physical activity is to combine them in a single workout. For example, a workout could begin with a warm-up consisting of flexibility exercises, followed by strength training exercises, and end with moderate-intensity aerobic activity.

In conclusion, different types of physical activity can provide different benefits for cancer prevention, and incorporating a variety of exercises into a comprehensive exercise plan can help reduce the risk of cancer. It is recommended to engage in at least 150 minutes of moderate-intensity aerobic activity per week, along with strength training exercises at least twice a week and flexibility exercises on a regular basis, but the specific exercise plan should be tailored to the individual's preferences, fitness level, and overall health status.

Strategies for Maintaining Regular Physical Activity

Maintaining regular physical activity can be challenging, as there are several common barriers that can make it difficult to stick to an exercise routine. These barriers include lack of time, lack of motivation, and physical limitations. However, there are several strategies that can help overcome these barriers and make physical activity a regular part of daily life.

One of the most effective strategies for making physical activity a regular part of daily life is to set goals. Setting realistic, achievable goals can provide motivation and help individuals stay on track with their exercise routine. Goals should be specific, measurable, and time-bound, such as aiming to walk for 30 minutes every day for the next month.

Tracking progress is another effective strategy for maintaining regular physical activity. Keeping a record of exercise sessions and tracking progress can provide a sense of accomplishment and motivation to continue. This can be done through a fitness app or journal.

Finding social support can also be helpful in maintaining regular physical activity. Exercising with a friend or joining a group fitness class can provide accountability and motivation. Additionally, social support can provide a sense of community and enjoyment, making physical activity more enjoyable.

Tailoring physical activity to individual needs and preferences is also important for maximum adherence and enjoyment. For example, some individuals may prefer to exercise in the morning, while others may prefer to exercise in the evening. Similarly, some individuals may prefer high-intensity workouts, while others may prefer low-intensity workouts such as yoga. It is important to find activities that are enjoyable and sustainable in the long-term.

Incorporating physical activity into daily life can also be done in small ways, such as taking the stairs instead of the elevator, parking further away from the store, or taking a short walk during a break at work.

In conclusion, common barriers to maintaining regular physical activity can be overcome through strategies such as setting goals, tracking progress, finding social support, tailoring physical activity to individual needs and preferences, and incorporating physical activity into daily life in small ways. By making physical activity a regular part of daily life, individuals can improve their overall health and reduce the risk of cancer and other chronic diseases.

Physical Activity and Cancer Survivorship

Physical activity can provide many benefits for cancer survivors, including reducing the risk of cancer recurrence and improving overall health and quality of life. Exercise can help to reduce inflammation, improve immune function, and promote healthy hormone levels, all of which can reduce the risk of cancer recurrence.

In addition to reducing the risk of cancer recurrence, physical activity can also improve overall health and quality of life for cancer survivors. Regular exercise can help to improve cardiovascular health, reduce fatigue, improve mood, and promote healthy weight management. Additionally, exercise can improve physical function and reduce the risk of chronic conditions such as osteoporosis and diabetes.

When it comes to physical activity guidelines for cancer survivors, it is important to work with healthcare professionals to develop an appropriate exercise plan. Cancer survivors may have unique physical and emotional challenges that require a tailored approach to physical activity. Healthcare professionals can help to develop an exercise plan that takes into account any physical limitations, medications, and other health conditions.

The American College of Sports Medicine (ACSM) has developed specific physical activity guidelines for cancer survivors. These guidelines recommend that cancer survivors engage in at least 150 minutes of moderate-intensity aerobic exercise per week, as well as at least two days of strength training per week. However, it is important to note that these guidelines may need to be modified based on individual needs and limitations.

In addition to the physical benefits, physical activity can also support the emotional challenges of cancer survivorship. Exercise can help to reduce anxiety and depression, improve self-esteem and body image, and provide a sense of control and empowerment. Additionally, participating in physical activity with others can provide social support and a sense of community.

In conclusion, physical activity can provide many benefits for cancer survivors, including reducing the risk of cancer recurrence and improving overall health and quality of life. It is important for cancer survivors to work with healthcare professionals to develop an appropriate exercise plan that takes into account their unique physical and emotional challenges. By incorporating physical activity into their daily routine, cancer survivors can improve their physical and emotional well-being and reduce the risk of chronic diseases.

Chapter 4:

Environmental Factors and Cancer Prevention

Environmental factors have been identified as significant contributors to cancer development. These factors include exposure to chemicals, air pollution, radiation, lifestyle choices, and diet. In this response, we will focus on exposure to chemicals, air pollution, and radiation.

Exposure to Chemicals: Many chemicals have been identified as carcinogenic or cancer-causing. Some examples of chemicals that have been linked to cancer include benzene, asbestos, arsenic, and formaldehyde. These chemicals are found in various products such as plastics, cleaning products, and building materials. Exposure to these chemicals can occur through inhalation, ingestion, or absorption through the skin.

Air Pollution: Air pollution is another environmental factor that has been linked to cancer. Studies have shown that exposure to air pollution increases the risk of lung cancer, as well as other types of cancer such as bladder and breast cancer. Air pollution can contain various toxins such as polycyclic aromatic hydrocarbons (PAHs), nitrogen oxides (NOx), and particulate matter (PM) which can enter the body through inhalation.

Radiation: Exposure to radiation is also a known environmental risk factor for cancer. High levels of exposure to ionizing radiation can cause DNA damage and increase the risk of cancer development. This type of radiation is found in various sources such as X-rays, gamma rays, and radioactive substances.

How Environmental Factors Can Damage DNA and Increase Cancer Risk:

DNA damage is a significant contributor to the development of cancer. Exposure to environmental factors such as chemicals, air pollution, and radiation can cause DNA damage in different ways. For example, chemicals such as benzene can bind to DNA, causing structural damage that can lead to mutations. Similarly, exposure to air pollution can lead to the formation of reactive oxygen species (ROS), which can cause oxidative DNA damage. Radiation exposure can also cause direct DNA damage by breaking the chemical bonds that hold DNA strands together.

When DNA damage occurs, it can result in mutations that can disrupt normal cellular functions, including the regulation of cell growth and division. Uncontrolled cell growth can lead to the development of cancer.

Challenges Associated with Identifying and Reducing Environmental Exposures that Contribute to Cancer Risk:

Identifying and reducing environmental exposures that contribute to cancer risk can be challenging. One of the biggest challenges is the sheer number of chemicals and pollutants that people are exposed to daily. It is estimated that there are over 80,000 chemicals used in various products, and only a small fraction of them have been thoroughly tested for their potential carcinogenic effects.

Additionally, the effects of environmental exposures on cancer risk can be cumulative and occur over long periods, making it challenging to pinpoint the specific factors responsible for cancer development. This complexity also makes it difficult to establish cause-and-effect relationships between environmental exposures and cancer development.

Another challenge is the lack of regulations and policies to control exposure to potentially harmful substances. Even when substances are identified as carcinogenic, the process of regulating and reducing exposure can be slow and challenging.

Overall, identifying and reducing environmental exposures that contribute to cancer risk require a multidisciplinary approach that involves cooperation between researchers, policymakers, and industries. It is also essential to prioritize public education and awareness about the potential risks of environmental exposures and the steps that individuals can take to reduce their exposure.

Chemicals and Cancer Risk

There are various chemicals that have been linked to increased cancer risk. Some of the most commonly studied chemicals include pesticides, herbicides, and industrial chemicals such as benzene, vinyl chloride, and formaldehyde.

Pesticides and herbicides: These chemicals are commonly used in agriculture to control pests and weeds. Studies have shown that exposure to pesticides and herbicides can increase the risk of several types of cancer, including non-Hodgkin's lymphoma, leukemia, and prostate cancer. Some examples of commonly used pesticides and herbicides include glyphosate, atrazine, and chlorpyrifos.

Industrial chemicals: Benzene, vinyl chloride, and formaldehyde are some examples of industrial chemicals that have been linked to cancer. Benzene is used in the production of various products such as plastics, synthetic fibers, and rubber. Exposure to benzene has been linked to leukemia and other types of cancer. Vinyl chloride is used in the production of plastics and has been linked to liver cancer. Formaldehyde is used in various building materials and household products and has been linked to nasopharyngeal cancer.

How Exposure to These Chemicals Can Occur:

Exposure to these chemicals can occur through occupational or environmental exposure, as well as through food, water, and household products.

Occupational exposure: Workers in various industries such as agriculture, manufacturing, and construction are at increased risk of exposure to pesticides, herbicides, and industrial chemicals.

Exposure can occur through inhalation, skin contact, or ingestion.

Environmental exposure: Exposure to these chemicals can also occur through environmental contamination, such as air and water pollution. For example, pesticides and herbicides can leach into groundwater and contaminate drinking water sources.

Food and water: Pesticides and herbicides can also be present in food and water. Residues of these chemicals can remain on fruits and vegetables, even after washing. Similarly, industrial chemicals can also contaminate food and water sources.

Household products: Formaldehyde, for example, can be present in various household products such as cleaning agents, cosmetics, and textiles. Exposure to formaldehyde can occur through inhalation or skin contact.

Overview of Strategies for Reducing Exposure to These Chemicals:

Reducing exposure to these chemicals can be challenging, but there are several strategies that individuals can implement to minimize their exposure.

Choose organic foods: Choosing organic foods can reduce exposure to pesticides and herbicides. Organic foods are grown without the use of synthetic pesticides and herbicides, reducing the risk of exposure.

Avoid pesticides and herbicides: Limiting or avoiding the use of pesticides and herbicides in the home and garden can also reduce exposure.

Use safer household products: Using safer household products that do not contain harmful chemicals such as formaldehyde can reduce exposure. Consumers can look for products that are labeled as "green" or "non-toxic."

Reduce occupational exposure: Employers can take measures to reduce exposure to these chemicals in the workplace. This can include providing protective equipment and limiting exposure time.

Reduce environmental exposure: Communities can work to reduce environmental contamination by limiting the use of pesticides and herbicides, and regulating industrial practices.

Overall, reducing exposure to these chemicals requires a combination of individual actions and broader policy changes. By implementing these strategies, individuals can minimize their exposure to these chemicals and reduce their risk of developing cancer.

Air Pollution and Cancer Risk

Air pollution has been linked to an increased risk of several types of cancer, including lung cancer. Air pollution is made up of a complex mixture of particles and gases, including nitrogen oxides, sulfur dioxide, ozone, and particulate matter. These pollutants can damage the lungs and increase the risk of cancer development.

Particulate matter, in particular, has been shown to be a significant contributor to lung cancer risk. These tiny particles can penetrate deep into the lungs, causing inflammation and damage to lung tissue. Over time, this damage can lead to the development of cancer.

Common Sources of Air Pollution:

There are various sources of air pollution, both indoors and outdoors. Some of the most common sources include:

Vehicle exhaust: Cars, trucks, and other vehicles emit pollutants such as nitrogen oxides and particulate matter, contributing to outdoor air pollution.

Industrial emissions: Manufacturing facilities, power plants, and other industrial sources can emit pollutants such as sulfur dioxide and particulate matter, contributing to outdoor air pollution.

Wood-burning stoves: Burning wood for heating or cooking can release particulate matter and other pollutants into the air, contributing to indoor air pollution.

Tobacco smoke: Smoking and exposure to secondhand smoke can release carcinogenic pollutants into the air, increasing the risk of lung cancer.

Overview of Strategies for Reducing Exposure to Air Pollution:

Reducing exposure to air pollution can be challenging, but there are several strategies that individuals can implement to minimize their exposure.

Use public transportation: Using public transportation can reduce the number of vehicles on the road and, in turn, reduce outdoor air pollution.

Avoid high-traffic areas: Avoiding high-traffic areas, such as busy highways, can reduce exposure to vehicle exhaust and other outdoor pollutants.

Improve indoor air quality: Improving indoor air quality by using air purifiers, reducing the use of wood-burning stoves, and avoiding smoking can reduce exposure to indoor air pollutants.

Support policies to reduce air pollution: Supporting policies such as increased regulations on industrial emissions and clean energy initiatives can help reduce outdoor air pollution.

In summary, exposure to air pollution has been linked to an increased risk of lung cancer and other types of cancer. Common sources of air pollution include vehicle exhaust, industrial emissions, and wood-burning stoves. Strategies for reducing exposure to air pollution include using public transportation, avoiding high-traffic areas, improving indoor air quality, and supporting policies to reduce air pollution. By implementing these strategies, individuals can minimize their exposure to air pollution and reduce their risk of developing cancer.

Radiation and Cancer Risk

Exposure to radiation can increase the risk of cancer development. There are two types of radiation that can be harmful to human health: ionizing radiation and non-ionizing radiation.

Ionizing radiation, which includes X-rays, CT scans, and radiation therapy, can cause damage to the DNA in cells. This damage can disrupt the normal functioning of the cell and increase the risk of cancer development. Non-ionizing radiation, such as radio waves from cell phones and other electronic devices, does not have enough energy to damage DNA directly. However, prolonged exposure to this type of radiation can still have biological effects that may increase cancer risk.

Common sources of ionizing radiation exposure include medical imaging tests and radiation therapy for cancer treatment. Non-ionizing radiation exposure is often associated with the use of cell phones and other electronic devices.

Strategies for Reducing Exposure to Radiation:

Reducing exposure to radiation can be challenging, but there are several strategies that individuals can implement to minimize their exposure.

Minimize unnecessary medical imaging tests: When possible, individuals should avoid unnecessary medical imaging tests, such as CT scans and X-rays. If a medical imaging test is necessary, individuals should discuss the risks and benefits with their healthcare provider and request the lowest possible radiation dose.

Use hands-free devices for cell phones: To reduce non-ionizing radiation exposure from cell phones, individuals can use hands-free devices, such as Bluetooth earpieces or speakerphones, instead of holding the phone directly against their head.

Limit exposure to radiation sources in the workplace: For individuals who work in jobs that involve exposure to radiation, such as nuclear power plant workers, it is important to follow proper safety procedures and limit exposure to radiation sources.

Be mindful of exposure to natural radiation sources: Natural sources of radiation, such as radon gas and cosmic radiation, can also increase cancer risk. Individuals should be aware of these sources and take steps to reduce exposure, such as testing homes for radon gas and limiting exposure to cosmic radiation during air travel.

In summary, exposure to radiation, both ionizing and non-ionizing, can increase the risk of cancer development. Strategies for reducing exposure to radiation include minimizing unnecessary medical imaging tests, using hands-free devices for cell phones, limiting exposure to radiation sources in the workplace, and being mindful of exposure to natural sources of radiation. By implementing these strategies, individuals can minimize their exposure to radiation and reduce their risk of developing cancer.

Practical Strategies for Reducing Environmental Exposures and Lowering Cancer Risk

Reducing exposure to environmental factors that can increase cancer risk can be challenging, but there are several steps individuals can take to incorporate these principles into their daily lives. Some of these steps include:

1. Eating organic foods and avoiding foods with high levels of pesticides and herbicides.
2. Using safer household cleaning and personal care products.

3. Filtering tap water or drinking bottled water that has been tested for contaminants.
4. Using public transportation, biking, or walking instead of driving alone.
5. Improving indoor air quality by using air filters and avoiding smoking and burning candles or incense.

Using Resources to Identify and Avoid Environmental Exposures:

There are many resources available to help individuals identify and avoid potential environmental exposures. The Environmental Working Group provides consumer guides on food, cleaning products, personal care products, and other household items that can help individuals make informed choices about what products they use. The National Institute of Environmental Health Sciences also provides information on potential environmental exposures and their health effects.

Advocating for Policies and Regulations:

Individual actions can only go so far in reducing environmental exposures. It is also important to advocate for policies and regulations that protect public health and reduce environmental exposures. This can involve supporting organizations that work on environmental issues, contacting elected officials to voice concerns about environmental policies, and supporting initiatives that promote sustainable and environmentally friendly practices.

Policies and regulations can have a significant impact on reducing environmental exposures. For example, regulations on air pollution from vehicles and industry can reduce exposure to harmful pollutants that can increase cancer risk. Policies promoting sustainable agriculture practices can reduce the use of pesticides and herbicides, reducing exposure to harmful chemicals. By advocating for policies and regulations that protect public health and reduce environmental exposures, individuals can have a broader impact on reducing cancer risk in their communities and beyond.

In summary, incorporating principles of reducing exposure to environmental factors into daily life can help individuals minimize their exposure to potential carcinogens. Resources such as the Environmental Working Group's consumer guides and the National Institute of Environmental Health Sciences can help individuals identify and avoid potential environmental exposures. Advocating for policies and regulations that protect public health and reduce environmental exposures is also important for reducing cancer risk at a broader level.

Chapter 5:

Lifestyle Factors and Cancer Prevention

Lifestyle Factors Linked to Increased Cancer Risk:

1. Diet: A diet high in processed and red meat, saturated and trans fats, and low in fiber, fruits, and vegetables, has been linked to an increased risk of certain cancers, including colorectal, breast, and prostate cancer.
2. Physical Activity: Lack of physical activity or a sedentary lifestyle has been linked to an increased risk of cancer. Regular exercise can help reduce the risk of colon, breast, and endometrial cancers.
3. Tobacco Use: Tobacco use is the leading cause of preventable cancer deaths. Smoking tobacco has been linked to lung, bladder, pancreatic, and other cancers.

4. Alcohol Use: Excessive alcohol consumption has been linked to an increased risk of various cancers, including breast, liver, and colorectal cancer.

5. Stress: Chronic stress can weaken the immune system and increase the risk of cancer. High levels of stress hormones, such as cortisol, can damage DNA and contribute to the development of cancer.

Overview of How These Lifestyle Factors Can Affect DNA and Increase the Risk of Cancer Development:

Cancer is a complex disease that involves the uncontrolled growth and division of abnormal cells. Lifestyle factors can affect DNA and increase the risk of cancer development in several ways:

1. Diet: A diet high in processed and red meat, saturated and trans fats, and

low in fiber, fruits, and vegetables, can lead to inflammation and oxidative stress, which can damage DNA and increase the risk of cancer.

2. Physical Activity: Regular exercise can help reduce inflammation and oxidative stress, which can help protect DNA from damage and reduce the risk of cancer.

3. Tobacco Use: Tobacco smoke contains carcinogens, which can damage DNA and cause mutations that lead to cancer.

4. Alcohol Use: Excessive alcohol consumption can lead to inflammation and oxidative stress, which can damage DNA and increase the risk of cancer.

5. Stress: Chronic stress can weaken the immune system and increase inflammation, which can damage DNA and increase the risk of cancer.

Challenges Associated with Changing Unhealthy Lifestyle Habits and Adopting Healthy Ones:

Changing unhealthy lifestyle habits and adopting healthy ones can be challenging. Some of the challenges include:

Lack of Awareness: Many people may not be aware of the link between lifestyle factors and cancer, which can make it difficult to motivate them to make lifestyle changes.

Availability and Accessibility of Healthy Options: Healthy food options may not be as readily available or affordable in some communities, which can make it difficult for individuals to adopt healthier eating habits.

Addiction: Nicotine addiction from tobacco use and alcohol addiction can make it difficult for individuals to quit these unhealthy habits.

Time Constraints: Busy schedules and work commitments may make it difficult for individuals to find time to exercise or prepare healthy meals.

Lack of Social Support: Lack of social support can make it difficult for individuals to make healthy lifestyle changes. It is essential to have supportive friends and family members who can provide motivation and encouragement.

In conclusion, adopting healthy lifestyle habits can significantly reduce the risk of cancer. However, changing unhealthy lifestyle habits can be challenging due to various factors, including addiction, lack of awareness, availability and accessibility of healthy options, time constraints, and lack of social support. It is essential to address these challenges to promote healthy lifestyle habits and reduce the risk of cancer.

Diet and Cancer Risk

Specific Dietary Factors Linked to Increased or Decreased Cancer Risk:

<u>Red and Processed Meats:</u> Eating red and processed meats has been linked to an increased risk of colorectal, pancreatic, and prostate cancers. Processed meats contain carcinogenic compounds, including nitrites and nitrates, which can damage DNA.

<u>Fruits and Vegetables:</u> Eating a diet high in fruits and vegetables has been linked to a reduced risk of several types of cancer, including lung, breast, and colorectal cancer. Fruits and vegetables contain antioxidants and phytochemicals that can help protect DNA from damage.

<u>Alcohol:</u> Drinking alcohol has been linked to an increased risk of several types of cancer, including breast, liver, and colorectal cancer. Alcohol can damage DNA and

increase the production of harmful compounds that can lead to cancer.

How Nutrients and Compounds in Food Can Affect DNA and Cancer Risk:

Antioxidants: Antioxidants, such as vitamin C, vitamin E, and beta-carotene, can help protect DNA from damage by neutralizing free radicals, which can cause oxidative stress. Oxidative stress can damage DNA and increase the risk of cancer.

Phytochemicals: Phytochemicals, such as carotenoids, flavonoids, and phenolic acids, can help protect DNA from damage and reduce the risk of cancer. Phytochemicals have anti-inflammatory and antioxidant properties that can help prevent cancer.

Carbohydrates: Eating a diet high in refined carbohydrates, such as sugar and white flour, can lead to inflammation and insulin resistance, which can increase the risk of cancer. Whole grains contain fiber, which can help reduce the risk of colon cancer.

Overview of Strategies for Adopting a Healthy and Cancer-Protective Diet:

Eat a variety of fruits and vegetables: Eating a variety of fruits and vegetables can provide a range of nutrients and phytochemicals that can help protect against cancer.

Choose whole grains: Whole grains, such as brown rice, quinoa, and whole wheat bread, contain fiber, vitamins, and minerals that can help reduce the risk of cancer.

Limit processed and red meats: Processed and red meats contain carcinogenic compounds that can damage DNA and increase the risk of cancer. Choosing lean proteins, such as fish, poultry, and beans, can help reduce the risk of cancer.

Limit alcohol: Drinking alcohol can increase the risk of several types of cancer. Limiting alcohol consumption or avoiding it altogether can help reduce the risk of cancer.

Stay hydrated: Drinking plenty of water can help flush out toxins and reduce the risk of cancer.

In conclusion, adopting a healthy and cancer-protective diet can help reduce the risk of cancer. Certain nutrients and compounds in food, such as antioxidants and phytochemicals, can help protect DNA from damage and reduce the risk of cancer. Strategies for adopting a healthy diet include eating a variety of fruits and vegetables, choosing whole grains and lean proteins, limiting processed and red meats, limiting alcohol consumption, and staying hydrated.

Physical Activity and Cancer Risk

Physical activity has been shown to reduce the risk of several types of cancer by reducing inflammation, improving immune function, and regulating hormones. Inflammation can lead to DNA damage, which can increase the risk of cancer. Regular physical activity can help reduce chronic inflammation and protect against cancer. Exercise also helps to improve immune function by increasing the circulation of immune cells and improving their ability to identify and destroy cancer cells. Physical activity can also help regulate hormones that can increase the risk of cancer, such as estrogen and insulin.

Types and Amounts of Physical Activity Associated with Lower Cancer Risk:

Aerobic exercise and strength training have both been associated with lower cancer risk. Aerobic exercise, such as brisk walking, jogging, or cycling, can help improve cardiovascular health and reduce the risk of several types of cancer, including breast, colon, and lung cancer. Strength training, such as weightlifting or resistance band exercises, can help build muscle and increase bone density, which can reduce the risk of certain cancers, such as breast and colon cancer.

The American Cancer Society recommends at least 150 minutes of moderate-intensity or 75 minutes of vigorous-intensity aerobic exercise per week, along with strength training exercises at least two days per week.

Strategies for Incorporating Physical Activity into Daily Life:

Incorporating physical activity into daily life can be easy and enjoyable. Here are some strategies for incorporating physical activity into daily life:

Walk or bike to work: If possible, consider walking or biking to work. This can help increase daily physical activity and reduce the risk of cancer.

Take the stairs: Instead of taking the elevator, take the stairs whenever possible. This can help increase heart rate and improve cardiovascular health.

Participate in recreational activities: Participating in recreational activities, such as hiking, swimming, or dancing, can be a fun way to increase physical activity and reduce the risk of cancer.

Join a fitness class: Joining a fitness class, such as yoga or aerobics, can provide social support and motivation to maintain a regular exercise routine.

Take breaks throughout the day: Taking breaks throughout the day to stretch, walk around, or do some light exercises can help increase physical activity and reduce the risk of cancer.

In conclusion, physical activity can help reduce the risk of cancer by reducing inflammation, improving immune function, and regulating hormones. Aerobic exercise and strength training have both been associated with lower cancer risk. Strategies for incorporating physical activity into daily life include walking or biking to work, taking the stairs, participating in recreational activities, joining a fitness class, and taking breaks throughout the day to stretch and move. By adopting a regular physical activity routine, individuals can help reduce their risk of cancer and improve their overall health and wellbeing.

Tobacco and Alcohol Use and Cancer Risk

Tobacco use is a well-established risk factor for cancer, including lung, bladder, and pancreatic cancer. Tobacco smoke contains more than 70 known carcinogens, including polycyclic aromatic hydrocarbons (PAHs), nitrosamines, and benzene. These chemicals can damage DNA, cause mutations, and promote the growth of cancer cells. Tobacco smoke can also suppress the immune system, making it more difficult for the body to identify and destroy cancer cells.

Lung cancer is the most well-known cancer associated with tobacco use, accounting for about 85% of all lung cancer cases. Smoking is also a major risk factor for bladder cancer, with smokers being about four times more likely to develop the disease than nonsmokers. Pancreatic cancer is also linked to smoking, with smokers having a 20-30% increased risk of developing the disease.

Alcohol use has also been linked to an increased risk of certain types of cancer, including breast, liver, and colorectal cancer. Alcohol is a known carcinogen and can damage DNA, promote the growth of cancer cells, and increase levels of hormones that can contribute to cancer development. For example, alcohol can increase levels of estrogen, which is associated with an increased risk of breast cancer. Alcohol can also damage the liver, leading to cirrhosis and an increased risk of liver cancer.

Strategies for quitting smoking and reducing alcohol use:

Quitting smoking and reducing alcohol use can be challenging, but there are several strategies that can help:

Nicotine replacement therapy: Nicotine replacement therapy, such as nicotine patches, gum, or lozenges, can help reduce withdrawal symptoms and cravings associated with quitting smoking.

Counseling: Counseling can help individuals develop coping strategies, set goals, and build a support network to help them quit smoking or reduce alcohol use.

Support groups: Joining a support group, such as Nicotine Anonymous or Alcoholics Anonymous, can provide social support and motivation to quit smoking or reduce alcohol use.

Medications: There are several medications available that can help reduce cravings and withdrawal symptoms associated with quitting smoking or reducing alcohol use.

Limiting exposure to triggers: Avoiding situations that trigger cravings for cigarettes or alcohol, such as social events where alcohol is present, can help reduce the risk of relapse.

In conclusion, tobacco use is a well-established risk factor for cancer, including lung, bladder, and pancreatic cancer. Alcohol use has also been linked to an increased risk of certain types of cancer, including breast, liver, and colorectal cancer. Strategies for quitting smoking and reducing alcohol use include nicotine replacement therapy, counseling, support groups, medications, and limiting exposure to triggers. By adopting these strategies, individuals can help reduce their risk of cancer and improve their overall health and wellbeing.

Stress and Cancer Risk

Chronic stress can increase cancer risk by affecting immune function and hormone regulation. Stress triggers the release of stress hormones such as cortisol and adrenaline, which can suppress the immune system and cause inflammation, both of which can increase the risk of cancer. Chronic stress can also disrupt hormone regulation, which can contribute to cancer development. For example, stress can increase levels of estrogen, which is associated with an increased risk of breast cancer.

Strategies for managing stress include meditation, yoga, and other mind-body practices. These practices can help reduce stress by promoting relaxation, reducing muscle tension, and calming the mind. Meditation involves focusing the mind on a specific object or idea, such as the breath, to promote relaxation and reduce stress. Yoga combines physical postures, breathing exercises, and meditation to promote relaxation, flexibility, and strength.

Social support is also important for reducing stress and promoting overall health. Having a support network of family, friends, or a community can provide emotional support, practical assistance, and a sense of belonging. Studies have shown that social support can help reduce stress and improve health outcomes, including a reduced risk of cancer.

Maintaining a positive outlook on life is also important for reducing stress and promoting overall health. This involves cultivating a positive attitude, focusing on the present moment, and finding meaning and purpose in life. Positive thinking can help reduce stress and improve mood, which can improve overall health and wellbeing.

In conclusion, chronic stress can increase cancer risk by affecting immune function and hormone regulation. Strategies for managing stress include meditation, yoga, and other mind-body practices, as well as maintaining social support and a positive outlook on life. By adopting these strategies, individuals can help reduce their risk of cancer and improve their overall health and wellbeing.

Practical Strategies for Adopting a Cancer-Protective Lifestyle

Adopting and maintaining healthy lifestyle habits can be challenging, especially in the context of busy schedules and competing priorities. However, there are several strategies that can help individuals overcome these challenges and adopt a cancer-protective lifestyle.

One important strategy is to set specific, measurable, achievable, relevant, and time-bound (SMART) goals. For example, instead of setting a vague goal like "exercise more," a SMART goal would be "walk for 30 minutes at least three times per week." By setting specific goals, individuals can track their progress and stay motivated to make lasting lifestyle changes.

Another strategy is to prioritize healthy habits by incorporating them into daily routines. For example, instead of trying to find time for exercise, individuals can walk or bike to work, take the stairs instead of the elevator, or participate in active recreational activities with friends and family.

Accountability is also important for making lasting lifestyle changes. This can involve enlisting the support of a friend, family member, or healthcare provider to help track progress, provide encouragement, and hold individuals accountable for their goals.

Social support is also crucial for making lasting lifestyle changes. By surrounding themselves with supportive friends and family members, individuals can receive encouragement, motivation, and practical support in their efforts to adopt a healthy lifestyle. Social support can also help individuals overcome obstacles and make sustained changes over time.

Adopting and maintaining healthy lifestyle habits is crucial for reducing cancer risk and promoting overall health and wellbeing. Strategies for achieving this include setting SMART goals, incorporating healthy habits into daily routines, enlisting accountability partners, and seeking social support. By adopting these strategies, individuals can make lasting lifestyle changes and reduce their risk of cancer.

Chapter 6:

Screening and Early Detection of Cancer

Early detection of cancer is crucial for improving cancer outcomes and survival rates. When cancer is detected early, it is typically easier to treat, and the chances of a successful outcome are much higher. Early detection also means that the cancer has not had as much time to spread to other parts of the body, which can be more difficult to treat.

Studies have shown that cancer screening programs can significantly reduce mortality rates for several types of cancer. For example, the American Cancer Society estimates that mammography screening has contributed to a 40% reduction in breast cancer mortality since the 1980s. Similarly, screening programs for colorectal cancer have been shown to reduce mortality rates by up to 60%.

It's important to note that cancer screening tests are not perfect, and there is always a chance of false positives (when the test indicates the presence of cancer when there is none) or false negatives (when the test fails to detect cancer that is present). However, despite these limitations, cancer screening is still an essential tool for detecting cancer early and improving outcomes.

Overview of Cancer Screening Tests Available for Different Types of Cancer:

There are several cancer screening tests available for different types of cancer, including mammography, colonoscopy, and Pap tests.

Mammography: Mammography is a screening test for breast cancer that involves taking X-ray images of the breast tissue. It is recommended that women aged 50-74 years have a mammogram every two years. Women who are at higher risk of breast cancer may be advised to have more frequent screenings or to start screening at an earlier age.

Colonoscopy: Colonoscopy is a screening test for colorectal cancer that involves examining the inside of the colon and rectum with a camera. The test is typically recommended for people aged 50 years and older, although people at higher risk of colorectal cancer may be advised to start screening earlier.

Pap test: The Pap test is a screening test for cervical cancer that involves collecting cells from the cervix and examining them under a microscope. The test is recommended for women aged 21-65 years and is typically done every three years. Women who have had a hysterectomy or who have had the

HPV vaccine may not need to have a Pap test.

Benefits and Limitations of Cancer Screening:

The benefits of cancer screening include detecting cancer early when it is more treatable, reducing mortality rates, and improving overall health outcomes. However, there are also some limitations to cancer screening, including the potential for false positives and overdiagnosis.

False positives occur when the screening test indicates the presence of cancer when there is none. False positives can cause anxiety and stress for the person being screened, and they may lead to unnecessary follow-up tests or treatments.

Overdiagnosis occurs when the screening test detects cancer that is not harmful and would not have caused any symptoms or health problems if left untreated. Overdiagnosis can lead to unnecessary treatments, which can have negative side effects.

Despite these limitations, cancer screening is still an essential tool for detecting cancer early and improving outcomes. People should discuss their screening options with their healthcare provider to determine which tests are appropriate for them based on their age, gender, and risk factors for cancer.

Breast Cancer Screening

Breast cancer is a common type of cancer that affects women worldwide. Early detection of breast cancer is essential for better treatment outcomes and improved survival rates. There are several screening methods available for breast cancer, including mammography, MRI, and ultrasound.

Mammography: Mammography is the most common screening method for breast cancer. It uses low-dose X-rays to create images of the breast tissue. Mammography is effective at detecting breast cancer at an early stage, even before symptoms appear. It is recommended that women aged 50-74 years have a mammogram every two years. Women at higher risk of breast cancer may be advised to start screening at an earlier age or to have more frequent screenings.

MRI: Magnetic resonance imaging (MRI) is another screening method for breast cancer. It uses powerful magnets and radio waves to create detailed images of the breast tissue. MRI is more sensitive than mammography and is often recommended for women at high risk of breast cancer, such as those with a family history or those with certain genetic mutations. MRI is not typically used as a routine screening tool due to its cost and availability.

Ultrasound: Breast ultrasound uses high-frequency sound waves to create images of the breast tissue. It is often used in combination with mammography for women with dense breast tissue or for those with abnormal findings on a mammogram. Ultrasound is not recommended as a routine screening tool for breast cancer.

Current Recommendations for Breast Cancer Screening:

The American Cancer Society recommends that women with an average risk of breast cancer start screening at age 45 and continue to have mammograms every year until age 54. After that, women should have a mammogram every two years. Women at higher risk of breast cancer, such as those with a family history or certain genetic mutations, may need to start screening earlier or have more frequent screenings.

Pros and Cons of Alternative Breast Cancer Screening Methods:

There are some alternative breast cancer screening methods available, such as thermography and breast self-exams.

Thermography: Thermography is a screening method that uses heat-sensitive imaging to detect changes in breast tissue. It is marketed as a non-invasive, radiation-free alternative to mammography. However, there is no evidence to support its effectiveness as a breast cancer screening tool. The American Cancer Society does not recommend thermography as a replacement for mammography or other established screening methods.

Breast self-exams: Breast self-exams involve women examining their own breasts for any lumps, changes, or abnormalities. While breast self-exams can help women become familiar with their breast tissue, there is no evidence to suggest that they are effective at detecting breast cancer early. The American Cancer Society recommends that women do not rely solely on breast self-exams for breast cancer screening.

In summary, mammography is the most commonly used screening method for breast cancer. MRI may be recommended for women at high risk of breast cancer, while ultrasound is often used in combination with mammography for certain patients. It is important for women to discuss their screening options with their healthcare provider and follow the recommended screening guidelines. While alternative screening methods such as thermography and breast self-exams may seem appealing, there is no evidence to support their effectiveness in detecting breast cancer early.

Prostate Cancer Screening

Prostate cancer is a common type of cancer that affects men worldwide. Early detection of prostate cancer is essential for better treatment outcomes and improved survival rates. There are two main screening methods available for prostate cancer, including the prostate-specific antigen (PSA) blood test and digital rectal exam.

PSA blood test: The PSA blood test measures the level of PSA in a man's blood. PSA is a protein produced by the prostate gland, and elevated levels can indicate the presence of prostate cancer or other prostate-related conditions. However, the PSA blood test is not specific to prostate cancer and can produce false positives or false negatives.

Digital rectal exam: During a digital rectal exam, a healthcare provider inserts a gloved, lubricated finger into the rectum to feel for any abnormalities in the prostate gland. While this method is less sensitive than the PSA blood test, it can detect some cancers that may be missed by the blood test.

Controversies Surrounding Prostate Cancer Screening:

There is ongoing controversy surrounding prostate cancer screening, mainly due to the potential for overdiagnosis and over-treatment. Overdiagnosis occurs when a cancer is detected and treated, even though it would not have caused harm or death if left untreated. Over-treatment refers to the unnecessary treatment of non-aggressive cancers that would not have caused harm.

Current Recommendations for Prostate Cancer Screening:

The American Cancer Society recommends that men discuss prostate cancer screening with their healthcare provider starting at age 50 for those at average risk of developing prostate cancer. Men at higher risk, such as those with a family history, should discuss screening with their healthcare provider starting at age 45. Men at the highest risk, such as African American men or those with a family history of early-onset prostate cancer, should discuss screening with their healthcare provider starting at age 40.

The frequency of prostate cancer screening depends on a man's age and risk factors. For men with a PSA level below 2.5 ng/mL and no other risk factors, screening can be done every two years. For those with a PSA level between 2.5 and 4 ng/mL, screening should be done yearly. Men with a PSA level above 4 ng/mL should undergo further testing, such as a biopsy.

In summary, prostate cancer screening methods include the PSA blood test and digital rectal exam. While there is controversy surrounding prostate cancer screening due to the potential for overdiagnosis and over-treatment, it is important for men to discuss their screening options with their healthcare provider and follow the recommended screening guidelines based on their age and risk factors.

Colorectal Cancer Screening

Colorectal cancer is a common type of cancer that affects the colon or rectum. Early detection of colorectal cancer is essential for better treatment outcomes and improved survival rates. There are several screening methods available for colorectal cancer, including colonoscopy, fecal occult blood tests (FOBTs), and stool DNA tests.

Colonoscopy: During a colonoscopy, a healthcare provider uses a long, flexible tube with a camera at the end to examine the inside of the colon and rectum for any abnormal growths or polyps that could be cancerous or precancerous. If any polyps are found, they can be removed during the procedure, reducing the risk of cancer.

Fecal Occult Blood Tests (FOBTs): FOBTs detect blood in the stool, which can be a sign of colorectal cancer. This test involves collecting a small sample of stool and sending it to a lab for analysis. There are two types of FOBTs: guaiac-based FOBT (gFOBT) and fecal immunochemical test (FIT).

Stool DNA tests: Stool DNA tests are a newer screening option that detect changes in DNA that are associated with colorectal cancer or precancerous polyps. These tests are typically performed every three years.

Current Recommendations for Colorectal Cancer Screening:

The American Cancer Society recommends that people at average risk of developing colorectal cancer begin screening at age 45. The frequency of screening depends on the type of test used. For colonoscopies, screening should be done every 10 years if no polyps are found. If polyps are found, the frequency of screening will depend on the size, number, and type of polyps.

For FOBTs, screening should be done every year. For stool DNA tests, screening should be done every three years.

Pros and Cons of Alternative Colorectal Cancer Screening Methods:

Virtual Colonoscopy: Virtual colonoscopy, also known as CT colonography, uses a CT scan to create images of the colon and rectum. While it is less invasive than a traditional colonoscopy, it still requires bowel preparation and can miss small polyps or lesions.

Stool-Based Tests: Stool-based tests, such as FOBTs and stool DNA tests, are less invasive than a colonoscopy and do not require sedation. However, they can produce false-positive results, leading to unnecessary follow-up testing or procedures.

In summary, there are several screening methods available for colorectal cancer, including colonoscopy, FOBTs, and stool DNA tests. People at average risk of developing colorectal cancer should begin screening at age 45 and follow the recommended frequency of screening based on the type of test used. Alternative screening methods, such as virtual colonoscopy and stool-based tests, have their own pros and cons and should be discussed with a healthcare provider.

Cervical Cancer Screening

Cervical cancer screening aims to detect any abnormalities or precancerous changes in the cells of the cervix, which is the lower part of the uterus that connects to the vagina. The most commonly used screening methods are the Pap test and the HPV test.

The Pap test, also called a Pap smear, involves collecting cells from the surface of the cervix using a small brush or spatula. The collected cells are then examined under a microscope to check for any abnormal changes in their shape or size, which could be a sign of precancerous or cancerous cells.

The HPV test involves collecting cells from the cervix, similar to the Pap test. However, instead of looking for abnormal cells, the HPV test checks for the presence of high-risk strains of the human papillomavirus (HPV), which is the most common cause of cervical cancer.

The current recommendations for cervical cancer screening vary depending on a person's age and health history. The American Cancer Society recommends that individuals with a cervix should start getting Pap tests at age 25 and continue to get them every three years until age 65. Alternatively, individuals can opt for HPV testing alone every five years from age 25 to 65. For those between the ages of 21 and 24, the Pap test is recommended every three years. Women who have had a hysterectomy (removal of the uterus and cervix) and no history of cervical cancer or precancerous lesions, do not need to be screened for cervical cancer.

HPV vaccination is also an important strategy for reducing the risk of cervical cancer. The HPV vaccine protects against the high-risk strains of the virus that are most likely to cause cervical cancer. The CDC recommends that all children, regardless of gender, should get the HPV vaccine at age 11 or 12, but it can be given as early as age 9. It is also recommended for individuals up to age 26 who have not been vaccinated previously. The vaccine is most effective when given before exposure to HPV, which is why it is recommended at a young age. Vaccination, along with regular screening, can significantly reduce the risk of developing cervical cancer.

Skin Cancer Screening

Skin cancer is one of the most common types of cancer and early detection is key to successful treatment. Skin cancer screening involves checking the skin for any unusual changes or growths that may indicate the presence of skin cancer. There are several screening methods used, including skin exams and dermoscopy.

- Skin Exams:
A skin exam involves a visual inspection of the skin by a healthcare professional.

During the exam, the healthcare professional will examine the entire body, looking for any unusual moles or growths that may be indicative of skin cancer. The exam may also include checking the scalp, fingernails, and toenails.

- Dermoscopy:

Dermoscopy is a non-invasive imaging technique that allows healthcare professionals to examine the skin at a higher magnification. The technique involves using a special instrument called a dermoscope to examine the skin. The dermoscope allows healthcare professionals to see beneath the surface of the skin, which can help identify any suspicious growths that may not be visible with the naked eye.

Overview of Current Recommendations for Skin Cancer Screening:

The current recommendations for skin cancer screening vary depending on an individual's risk factors. For those at average risk, the American Academy of Dermatology recommends a full-body skin exam every three years starting at age 20, and a yearly exam for those over 40 years old. However, those at higher risk due to family history or a personal history of skin cancer may need more frequent screenings.

It is important to note that individuals should also regularly perform self-exams at home to check for any changes or growths on their skin. If any suspicious changes are noticed, they should be reported to a healthcare professional immediately.

Importance of Sun Protection for Preventing Skin Cancer:

Sun exposure is one of the primary risk factors for skin cancer. The harmful ultraviolet (UV) rays from the sun can cause damage to the skin, leading to the development of skin cancer. Therefore, it is important to take steps to protect the skin from sun exposure.

Some ways to protect the skin from sun exposure include:

- Wearing protective clothing, such as long-sleeved shirts and wide-brimmed hats
- Using sunscreen with a minimum SPF of 30 and reapplying every two hours or after swimming or sweating
- Avoiding sun exposure during peak hours, typically between 10 a.m. and 4 p.m.
- Seeking shade when possible, such as under an umbrella or tree

Taking steps to protect the skin from sun exposure can help prevent the development of skin cancer and is an important part of overall skin health.

Creating a Personalized Cancer Screening Plan

Cancer screening plans should be personalized based on individual risk factors and preferences. Some important risk factors to consider include family history, age, lifestyle factors such as smoking and diet, and exposure to environmental toxins. Personal preferences may also play a role in deciding which screening tests to pursue.

To create a personalized cancer screening plan, individuals should consult with their healthcare provider. The provider can assess individual risk factors and recommend appropriate screening tests based on current guidelines. It is important to discuss any concerns or questions about the recommended tests and to work collaboratively with the healthcare provider to determine the best screening plan.

Overview of Communicating with Healthcare Providers about Cancer Screening:

When communicating with healthcare providers about cancer screening, it is important to be prepared and informed. This includes understanding individual risk factors and preferences, as well as current screening guidelines. Some important points to consider when discussing cancer screening with a healthcare provider include:

- ☐ Being open and honest about personal health history and any concerns or questions about screening tests
- ☐ Asking about the risks and benefits of specific screening tests
- ☐ Understanding the limitations of screening tests and their potential to produce false positives or false negatives

☐ Discussing any discomfort or anxiety related to screening tests and exploring ways to minimize these feelings

☐ Working collaboratively with the healthcare provider to determine the most appropriate screening plan based on individual risk factors and preferences.

Importance of Follow-up and Continued Monitoring after Cancer Screening Tests:

Follow-up and continued monitoring after cancer screening tests are important for several reasons. First, if a screening test detects a potential problem, follow-up tests can help confirm or rule out the presence of cancer. Second, regular monitoring can help detect cancer at an earlier stage when it may be more treatable.

In addition to regular monitoring, individuals should be aware of potential signs and symptoms of cancer and report any concerns to their healthcare provider. It is also important to maintain a healthy lifestyle, including regular exercise and a balanced diet, which can help reduce the risk of cancer.

In conclusion, creating a personalized cancer screening plan based on individual risk factors and preferences is important for early detection and treatment of cancer. Communicating effectively with healthcare providers about screening tests and advocating for appropriate tests can help ensure that individuals receive the best possible care. Finally, continued monitoring and follow-up after screening tests are important for maintaining overall health and well-being.

Chapter 7:

Lifestyle Factors and Cancer Prevention

Lifestyle factors such as diet, physical activity, smoking, alcohol consumption, and exposure to environmental toxins are known to play a significant role in cancer risk.

Dietary factors can both increase or decrease the risk of cancer. A diet high in processed and red meats, saturated and trans fats, and sugar can increase the risk of cancer, particularly colorectal and breast cancer. In contrast, a diet high in fruits, vegetables, whole grains, and lean protein can help reduce the risk of cancer.

Physical activity has been linked to a lower risk of many types of cancer, including breast, colon, and lung cancer. Regular physical activity can also help manage weight and reduce inflammation in the body, which can further reduce cancer risk.

Smoking is a well-known risk factor for several types of cancer, including lung, bladder, and pancreatic cancer. Secondhand smoke exposure is also linked to an increased risk of cancer.

Excessive alcohol consumption is associated with an increased risk of several types of cancer, including breast, liver, and colorectal cancer. Even moderate alcohol consumption has been linked to an increased risk of breast cancer.

Exposure to environmental toxins such as asbestos, radon, and certain chemicals can also increase the risk of cancer. These toxins can damage DNA and other cellular processes, leading to the development of cancer.

Genetics and epigenetics can also play a role in cancer risk. Certain inherited gene mutations, such as those in the BRCA1 and

BRCA2 genes, are known to increase the risk of breast and ovarian cancer. However, inherited genetic mutations account for only a small percentage of all cancer cases.

Epigenetics refers to changes in gene expression that do not involve changes to the DNA sequence itself. These changes can be influenced by lifestyle factors such as diet and exposure to toxins, and can impact cancer risk. For example, exposure to environmental toxins can cause epigenetic changes that lead to an increased risk of cancer.

Overall, cancer risk is influenced by a combination of factors, including genetics, epigenetics, and lifestyle factors. By adopting a healthy lifestyle and avoiding exposure to known toxins, individuals can take steps to reduce their risk of cancer.

Diet and Cancer Prevention

A healthy diet that includes fruits, vegetables, whole grains, and lean proteins has been shown to reduce the risk of several types of cancer. These foods are rich in nutrients and antioxidants that help to protect against cancer by reducing inflammation, neutralizing free radicals, and supporting a healthy immune system.

On the other hand, consumption of processed and red meats, saturated and trans fats, and sugar-sweetened beverages has been linked to an increased risk of cancer. Processed and red meats contain high levels of saturated fat and heme iron, which can damage cells and increase the risk of colon, stomach, and pancreatic cancer. Saturated and trans fats, which are found in many processed and fast foods, can contribute to inflammation and increase the risk of several types of cancer, including breast and colon cancer. High consumption of sugar-sweetened beverages has been linked to an increased risk of several types of cancer, including breast and colon cancer.

To create a healthy and balanced diet that promotes cancer prevention, it is important to focus on nutrient-dense foods such as:

- Fruits and vegetables: aim for a variety of colors and types, and try to eat at least 5 servings per day.
- Whole grains: choose whole grain breads, pasta, and rice instead of refined grains, which have been linked to an increased risk of colon cancer.
- Lean proteins: choose lean sources of protein such as fish, chicken, beans, and legumes, and limit red and processed meats.
- Healthy fats: choose healthy sources of fats such as nuts, seeds, avocados, and olive oil, and limit saturated and trans fats.

In addition, it is important to limit or avoid:

- Processed and red meats: limit consumption of these meats and choose leaner cuts when possible.
- Saturated and trans fats: limit consumption of fried and processed foods, baked goods, and high-fat dairy products.
- Sugar-sweetened beverages: choose water or unsweetened beverages instead of soda, sports drinks, and fruit juices with added sugars.

Overall, a healthy and balanced diet that emphasizes fruits, vegetables, whole grains, and lean proteins can help to reduce the risk of cancer and support overall health and well-being.

Physical Activity and Cancer Prevention

Physical activity has been shown to reduce the risk of several types of cancer, including breast, colon, and lung cancer. The mechanisms by which physical activity reduces cancer risk are not fully understood, but research suggests that physical activity can help to reduce inflammation, improve immune function, and regulate hormones such as insulin and estrogen, all of which can contribute to the development of cancer.

Regular physical activity is also important for maintaining a healthy body weight, which is an important factor in reducing cancer risk. Physical activity can also improve cardiovascular health, reduce stress, and improve overall quality of life.

For cancer prevention, the American Cancer Society recommends at least 150 minutes of moderate-intensity or 75 minutes of vigorous-intensity aerobic activity per week, along with muscle-strengthening activities at least 2 days per week. Moderate-intensity activities include brisk walking, cycling, and swimming, while vigorous-intensity activities include running, aerobic dancing, and heavy yard work.

In addition to reducing cancer risk, physical activity has numerous other health benefits. Regular physical activity can help to improve cardiovascular health by reducing the risk of heart disease and stroke, as well as manage weight and improve mental health. Physical activity has also been shown to reduce the risk of type 2 diabetes, osteoporosis, and depression.

Overall, physical activity is an important component of a healthy lifestyle that can help to reduce the risk of cancer and improve overall health and well-being. By incorporating regular physical activity into daily life, individuals can take steps to reduce their cancer risk and improve their overall health.

Smoking and Cancer Prevention

Smoking is one of the leading causes of cancer and is responsible for around one-third of all cancer deaths. Smoking is a known risk factor for several types of cancer, including lung, throat, mouth, esophageal, pancreatic, bladder, kidney, and cervical cancer. When tobacco smoke is inhaled, it contains over 70 known carcinogens that can damage DNA and other genetic material in cells, leading to the development of cancer.

Lung cancer is the most common type of cancer associated with smoking, accounting for about 80% of all smoking-related cancer deaths. Smokers are about 15 to 30 times more likely to develop lung cancer than non-smokers. Smoking is also a major risk factor for other types of respiratory cancers, including throat, mouth, and esophageal cancer. In addition, smoking increases the risk of pancreatic cancer by 2-3 times and bladder cancer by 4-7 times.

Quitting smoking is the best way to reduce the risk of cancer and improve overall health. Even if an individual has smoked for many years, quitting can still reduce the risk of cancer and improve overall life expectancy. Within just a few months of quitting, the body begins to heal and repair the damage caused by smoking. Within 5 years of quitting, the risk of many types of cancer, including lung cancer, is cut in half.

There are several resources and strategies available to help individuals quit smoking, including nicotine replacement therapy (NRT) and behavioral interventions. Nicotine replacement therapy includes gum, patches, lozenges, inhalers, and nasal sprays that deliver nicotine to the body without the harmful chemicals found in cigarettes. Behavioral interventions can include counseling, support groups, and other forms of therapy to help individuals overcome the psychological and emotional aspects of addiction.

In addition to NRT and behavioral interventions, there are several other strategies that can be helpful in quitting smoking, such as avoiding triggers, finding healthy alternatives to smoking, and developing a strong support network. By using a combination of strategies and seeking support, individuals can increase their chances of successfully quitting smoking and reducing their cancer risk.

Alcohol Consumption and Cancer Prevention

Alcohol consumption is a known risk factor for several types of cancer, including breast, liver, colorectal, and esophageal cancer. When alcohol is consumed, it is broken down in the body into a substance called acetaldehyde, which is a known carcinogen that can damage DNA and other genetic material in cells, leading to the development of cancer.

Breast cancer is the most common type of cancer associated with alcohol consumption, and even moderate drinking can increase the risk. Studies have shown that women who consume just one alcoholic drink per day are about 5-9% more likely to develop breast cancer than women who do not drink alcohol. Alcohol consumption is also a risk factor for liver cancer, with heavy alcohol use being a major risk factor for the development of liver cirrhosis, which is a known precursor to liver cancer.

For cancer prevention, the American Cancer Society recommends that adults limit their alcohol consumption to no more than 1 drink per day for women and 2 drinks per day for men. A standard drink is defined as

12 ounces of beer, 5 ounces of wine, or 1.5 ounces of distilled spirits.

Strategies for reducing alcohol consumption can include setting limits on consumption, avoiding triggers, and finding healthy alternatives to alcohol. For example, individuals can try drinking non-alcoholic beverages, such as water or herbal tea, or engaging in activities that do not involve alcohol, such as exercise or spending time with friends and family. Additionally, seeking support from friends, family, or a professional can be helpful in reducing alcohol consumption.

It is important to note that while moderate alcohol consumption may have some health benefits, such as reducing the risk of heart disease, the risks associated with alcohol consumption, including the risk of cancer, outweigh the potential benefits. By limiting alcohol consumption and finding alternative ways to socialize and celebrate, individuals can take steps to reduce their cancer risk and improve their overall health.

Environmental Toxins and Cancer Prevention

Environmental toxins, including air pollution, pesticides, and chemicals in consumer products, have been linked to an increased risk of cancer. Exposure to these toxins can damage DNA and other genetic material in cells, leading to the development of cancer. Air pollution has been associated with lung cancer and other respiratory cancers, while exposure to pesticides has been linked to an increased risk of several types of cancer, including leukemia and lymphoma. Chemicals in consumer products, such as phthalates and bisphenol A (BPA), have also been linked to an increased risk of cancer, particularly breast cancer.

To reduce exposure to environmental toxins, individuals can take several steps, including choosing safer products and reducing exposure to air pollution. For example, individuals can choose products that are free of harmful chemicals and use natural cleaning products instead of harsh chemicals. They can also reduce exposure to air pollution by avoiding heavily trafficked areas during peak traffic hours, using air purifiers in their homes, and choosing to walk, bike, or use public transportation instead of driving a car.

Current regulations and policies around environmental toxins and cancer prevention vary by country and region. In the United States, the Environmental Protection Agency (EPA) is responsible for regulating environmental toxins, including air pollutants and pesticides. The EPA sets standards for the amount of pollutants that can be released into the air and water and regulates the use of pesticides in agriculture.

In addition, the Food and Drug Administration (FDA) regulates chemicals in consumer products, including cosmetics, and sets limits on the amount of certain chemicals that can be used.

Overall, reducing exposure to environmental toxins is an important step in cancer prevention. By choosing safer products and reducing exposure to air pollution, individuals can take proactive steps to reduce their cancer risk and improve their overall health.

Creating a Cancer-Preventive Lifestyle Plan

Integrating healthy lifestyle behaviors into daily life is key to reducing cancer risk. This includes maintaining a healthy diet, engaging in regular physical activity, avoiding tobacco and excessive alcohol consumption, and reducing exposure to environmental toxins. However, making significant lifestyle changes can be challenging, so it's important to set realistic goals and track progress towards a cancer-preventive lifestyle.

One way to set realistic goals is to start with small changes and gradually build up to larger ones. For example, if someone currently doesn't engage in any physical activity, they could start with a daily 10-minute walk and gradually increase the duration and intensity of their exercise. Similarly, someone who doesn't typically eat a lot of fruits and vegetables could start by incorporating one serving into their daily diet and gradually increase the amount over time.

Tracking progress can also be helpful for maintaining motivation and staying on track towards a cancer-preventive lifestyle. This can be done by keeping a journal, using a fitness app to track exercise and diet, or setting reminders for healthy habits throughout the day.

Additionally, having a support system can be crucial for maintaining a cancer-preventive lifestyle. This could include enlisting the help of family and friends, joining a support group or fitness class, or working with a healthcare professional or registered dietitian to develop a personalized plan and receive guidance and support.

In summary, integrating healthy lifestyle behaviors into daily life to reduce cancer risk involves setting realistic goals, tracking progress, and maintaining motivation and support. By making small, sustainable changes and enlisting the help of others, individuals can take proactive steps towards a healthier, cancer-preventive lifestyle.

Chapter 8:

Cancer Screening and Early Detection

Early detection of cancer is critical for improving outcomes and increasing survival rates. When cancer is detected early, it is more likely to be treatable and potentially curable. In contrast, when cancer is diagnosed at a later stage, it may have already spread to other parts of the body, making it more difficult to treat and reducing the chances of survival.

There are several different types of cancer screening tests available, and recommendations for when and how often to undergo screening may vary based on factors such as age, family history, and other individual risk factors. Some of the most common cancer screening tests include:

Mammography: A type of X-ray that is used to screen for breast cancer. Recommendations for mammography screening may vary depending on individual risk factors, but in general, women are recommended to begin regular mammography screening at age 50 and continue every two years until age 74.

Pap test: A test used to screen for cervical cancer by detecting abnormal cells in the cervix. The recommended frequency of Pap testing may vary depending on individual risk factors, but in general, women are recommended to begin regular Pap testing at age 21 and continue every three years until age 65.

Colonoscopy: A test used to screen for colon cancer by examining the colon and rectum for abnormal growths or polyps. Recommendations for colonoscopy screening may vary depending on individual risk factors, but in general, individuals are recommended to begin regular colonoscopy screening at age 45 or earlier if they have certain risk factors.

Prostate-specific antigen (PSA) test: A blood test used to screen for prostate cancer. Recommendations for PSA testing may vary depending on individual risk factors, but in general, men are recommended to discuss the potential benefits and limitations of PSA testing with their healthcare provider starting at age 50 or earlier if they have certain risk factors.

While cancer screening tests can be valuable tools for early detection, they are not without limitations. False positives, where a screening test indicates the presence of cancer when none is actually present, can occur, leading to unnecessary anxiety and follow-up testing. Overdiagnosis, where a screening test detects a cancer that would not have caused harm during a person's lifetime, can also occur, leading to unnecessary treatment and potential harm.

In summary, early detection of cancer is critical for improving outcomes and survival rates. Cancer screening tests are an important tool for detecting cancer early, but they are not without limitations. Individuals should discuss the potential benefits and limitations of cancer screening with their healthcare provider to determine the most appropriate screening plan based on individual risk factors.

Section Breast Cancer Screening

Breast cancer screening is the process of looking for breast cancer before any symptoms develop. There are several types of breast cancer screening tests, including mammography, clinical breast exam, and breast MRI.

Mammography is the most commonly used screening test for breast cancer. It uses X-rays to create images of the breast tissue. During a mammogram, the breast is compressed between two plates, which can be uncomfortable for some women. Mammograms are most effective at detecting breast cancer in women over the age of 50, but they can also be used for women between the ages of 40 and 50, depending on individual risk factors.

A clinical breast exam is a physical exam performed by a healthcare provider to check for lumps or other changes in the breast tissue. This exam may also include a check of the lymph nodes in the armpit. Clinical breast exams may be performed as part of a routine physical exam or in response to symptoms.

Breast MRI is a screening test that uses a magnetic field and radio waves to create detailed images of the breast tissue. It is usually recommended for women who have a high risk of developing breast cancer due to factors such as a strong family history or a genetic mutation.

The recommended breast cancer screening guidelines may vary depending on an individual's age and risk factors. In general, the American Cancer Society recommends that women at average risk of developing breast cancer begin annual mammograms at age 45 and transition to mammograms every two years at age 55. Women between the ages of 40 and 44 may choose to begin annual mammograms if they wish, while women over the age of 55 may choose to continue annual mammograms if they prefer.

For women at higher risk of developing breast cancer due to factors such as a strong family history or a genetic mutation, earlier or more frequent screening may be recommended. This may include a combination of mammography, clinical breast exam, and breast MRI.

There are several risk factors that may affect breast cancer screening recommendations. These may include personal or family history of breast cancer, genetic mutations such as BRCA1 or BRCA2, and previous radiation therapy to the chest. Women who are at higher risk of developing breast cancer may benefit from earlier or more frequent screening to increase the chances of detecting cancer at an early stage.

In summary, breast cancer screening tests including mammography, clinical breast exam, and breast MRI are important tools for detecting breast cancer early. Recommended screening guidelines may vary depending on an individual's age and risk factors, and healthcare providers can work with patients to determine the most appropriate screening plan based on individual risk factors.

Colorectal Cancer Screening

Colorectal cancer screening tests are recommended for individuals who are at average risk or high risk of developing colorectal cancer. For individuals at average risk, screening is usually recommended to begin at age 45 or 50, while for those at higher risk, screening may be recommended to begin earlier or be more frequent.

There are several different types of colorectal cancer screening tests, including:

Colonoscopy: A colonoscopy is a procedure that uses a long, flexible tube with a camera at the end to examine the inside of the colon and rectum. During the procedure, the doctor can remove any polyps or abnormal tissue for further testing. Colonoscopies are generally recommended every 10 years starting at age 45 or 50 for individuals at average risk.

Fecal occult blood test (FOBT): An FOBT is a test that checks for hidden blood in the stool, which can be a sign of colorectal cancer. The test is done at home by collecting a stool sample and sending it to a lab for analysis. FOBTs are generally recommended every year starting at age 45 or 50 for individuals at average risk.

Stool DNA test: A stool DNA test is a newer type of screening test that looks for changes in DNA that can indicate the presence of cancer or precancerous growths in the colon. The test is done at home by collecting a stool sample and sending it to a lab for analysis. Stool DNA tests are generally recommended every 3 years starting at age 45 or 50 for individuals at average risk.

Other screening tests, such as flexible sigmoidoscopy, virtual colonoscopy, and double-contrast barium enema, may also be used in certain situations.

Factors that can increase an individual's risk of developing colorectal cancer include age, a personal history of colorectal polyps or cancer, a family history of colorectal cancer, a history of inflammatory bowel disease, and certain genetic syndromes. Depending on these risk factors, individuals may be recommended to start screening earlier or have more frequent screening tests. It is important to discuss your individual risk factors and screening recommendations with your healthcare provider.

Lung Cancer Screening

Early detection is critical for improving lung cancer outcomes and survival rates. Unfortunately, lung cancer often does not cause symptoms in its early stages, making it difficult to detect until it has progressed to more advanced stages. This is why screening for lung cancer is so important, especially in individuals at high risk for the disease.

The most common screening test for lung cancer is a low-dose computed tomography (LDCT) scan. This type of scan uses a small amount of radiation to create detailed images of the lungs. LDCT scans can detect small nodules or masses in the lungs that may be cancerous, even before symptoms appear. However, LDCT scans are not perfect and can still miss some early-stage cancers, while also identifying benign nodules that could lead to further testing and procedures.

Current guidelines recommend annual LDCT screening for individuals who are at high risk for lung cancer due to their smoking history or other risk factors. This includes individuals aged 50-80 years who have smoked the equivalent of one pack of cigarettes per day for at least 20 years, or those who have quit smoking within the past 15 years.

While LDCT screening has the potential to reduce lung cancer deaths by detecting the disease earlier, it also has limitations. One of the main limitations is that it can produce false positive results, which means that a scan may identify a nodule or mass that is not cancerous, but that requires further testing and procedures to confirm. Additionally, LDCT screening can also lead to overdiagnosis, which means that some individuals may be diagnosed and treated for cancers that would not have caused harm if left untreated.

Therefore, it is important for individuals who undergo LDCT screening to have follow-up care and discussion with their healthcare provider regarding the results, interpretation and any necessary actions. Additionally, the best way to reduce lung cancer risk is to quit smoking or avoid tobacco products altogether.

Prostate Cancer Screening

Prostate cancer screening tests primarily include a prostate-specific antigen (PSA) blood test and a digital rectal exam (DRE). The PSA test measures the levels of a protein produced by the prostate gland in the blood. Elevated PSA levels may indicate the presence of prostate cancer or other non-cancerous conditions like an enlarged prostate or prostate inflammation. A DRE involves a doctor or healthcare provider inserting a gloved, lubricated finger into the rectum to feel for any abnormalities in the prostate gland.

There is ongoing controversy over the benefits and potential harms of prostate cancer screening, particularly with the PSA test. The PSA test may lead to overdiagnosis and overtreatment of prostate cancer, as elevated PSA levels may not necessarily indicate the presence of cancer, and some prostate cancers may never become life-threatening. Additionally, prostate cancer treatments like surgery and radiation therapy can have significant side effects like impotence and urinary incontinence.

Current guidelines recommend that men discuss the potential benefits and harms of prostate cancer screening with their healthcare providers, especially if they are at higher risk due to factors such as age, family history, or race. For men with an average risk of prostate cancer, the United States Preventive Services Task Force recommends that screening with the PSA test should be an individual decision made after discussing potential benefits and harms with their healthcare provider starting at age 50. For men at higher risk, such as those with a family history of prostate cancer or African American men, screening discussions should start at age 45. The frequency of screening may vary based on individual risk factors and test results.

Prostate cancer risk factors include age, family history of prostate cancer, race (African American men are at higher risk), and certain genetic mutations. Men with a higher risk of prostate cancer may be recommended for earlier or more frequent screening. However, it is important to weigh the potential benefits and harms of screening on a case-by-case basis, taking into account individual risk factors and personal preferences.

Skin Cancer Screening

Skin cancer screening aims to detect skin cancer early when it is most treatable. The screening process usually involves a visual skin examination, which can be done by a healthcare professional or performed at home by oneself. In addition, dermoscopy is another screening test that is commonly used by dermatologists to examine suspicious moles or lesions.

For individuals at high risk of skin cancer due to sun exposure or other risk factors such as a personal or family history of skin cancer, fair skin, or a weakened immune system, it is recommended to have a full-body skin examination annually by a healthcare professional. The American Academy of Dermatology also recommends monthly self-exams to check for new or changing moles or lesions.

Reducing the risk of skin cancer involves protecting the skin from sun damage. This includes wearing protective clothing, such as hats and long-sleeved shirts, seeking shade, and applying a broad-spectrum sunscreen with an SPF of 30 or higher. It is also important to avoid indoor tanning, as this increases the risk of skin cancer.

Early detection and prompt treatment of skin cancer is crucial for a positive outcome. If a suspicious mole or lesion is identified during a skin examination, a biopsy may be necessary to confirm the diagnosis. If skin cancer is detected, treatment options may include surgery, radiation therapy, and chemotherapy, depending on the type and stage of cancer.

Other Cancer Screening Tests

In addition to breast, colorectal, lung, and skin cancer screening, there are other types of cancer screening tests available.

Cervical cancer screening typically involves a Pap test or an HPV test, or a combination of both. The recommended age to start cervical cancer screening is 21, and the frequency of screening depends on the screening method and the woman's age and risk factors.

Prostate cancer screening typically involves a prostate-specific antigen (PSA) blood test and a digital rectal exam (DRE). The recommended age to start prostate cancer screening and the frequency of screening depend on the man's age, risk factors, and personal preferences.

The recommended screening guidelines for each type of cancer vary depending on a person's age, gender, and risk factors. It is important to consult with a healthcare provider to determine the appropriate screening schedule.

Making Informed Decisions About Cancer Screening

Informed decision-making is an important aspect of cancer screening. While cancer screening tests can offer potential benefits, they can also have risks, including false-positive results, overdiagnosis, overtreatment, and anxiety. Therefore, it is important to understand the potential benefits and risks of screening tests and make informed decisions about cancer screening based on individual preferences and values.

To make an informed decision about cancer screening, it is important to weigh the potential benefits and risks of the test. Benefits can include the early detection and treatment of cancer, which can improve outcomes and survival rates. Risks can include false-positive results, overdiagnosis, overtreatment, and anxiety. It is also important to consider personal factors, such as age, family history, and overall health, when making decisions about cancer screening.

Healthcare providers play an important role in providing information and guidance about cancer screening decisions. They can help individuals understand their risk for cancer, explain the benefits and risks of screening tests, and provide guidance on how to make an informed decision. It is important for individuals to have open and honest communication with their healthcare provider to ensure that they are making the best decision for their individual circumstances.